Max and Mandi:
The Hippos with Human Teeth

Michael T. Nykamp

DEDICATION

To
Cora Jo
Avery Jean
Lynlee Kay

ACKNOWLEDGMENTS

Thank you to all who helped make this dream a reality. You know who you are.

Max and Mandi Boans were just like any other hippos.

They ate like hippos; they bathed like hippos; they talked like hippos.

They even went to school like hippos.

There was one odd thing about Max and Mandi, however. They did not brush their teeth like hippos.

You see, Max and Mandi did not have hippo teeth. They had people teeth, like you and me.

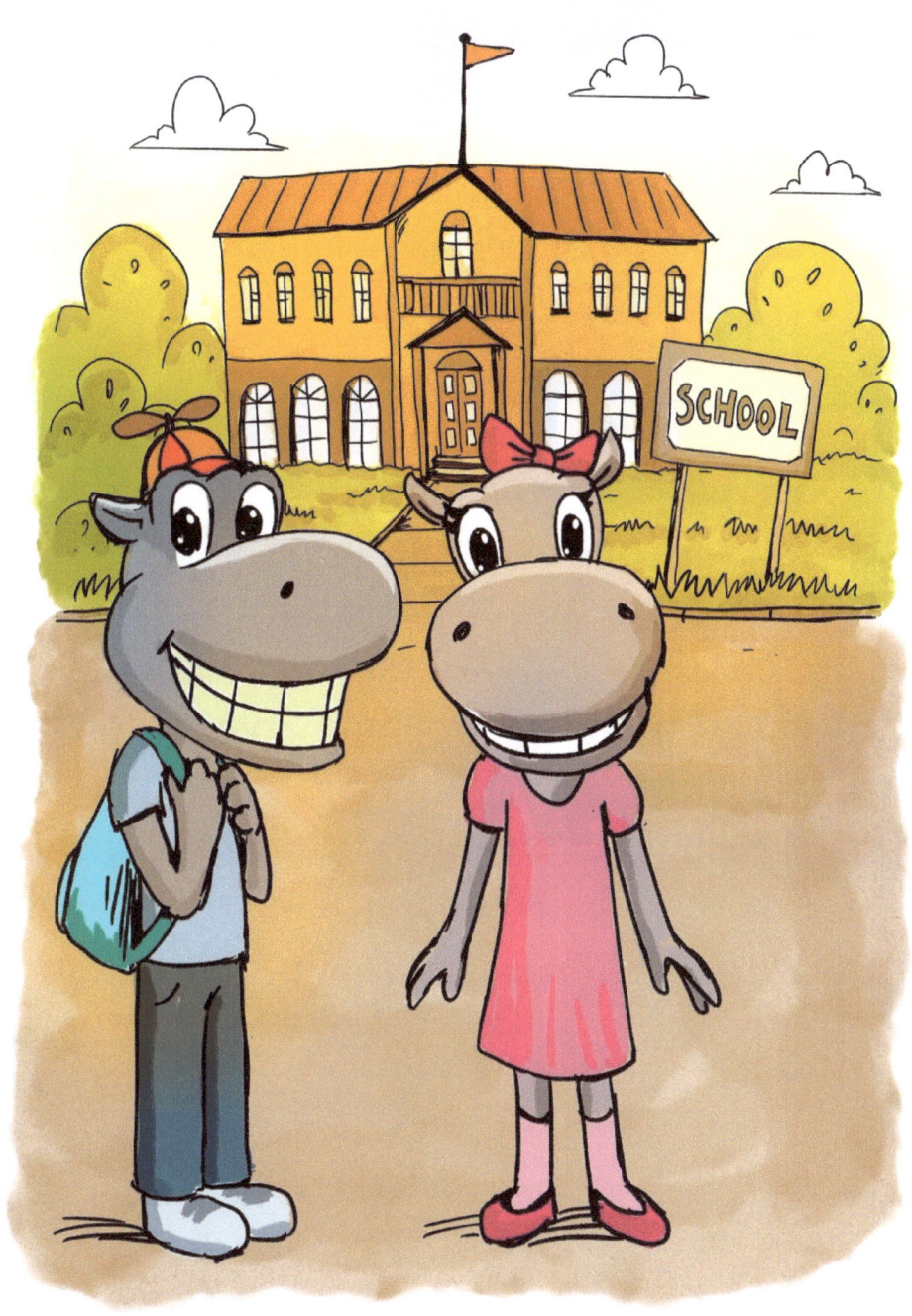

Mandi was incredibly proud of her human teeth. Every night before going to bed and every morning after waking up, she would brush her beautiful teeth while humming a tune.

Hmm Hmmmmmmmm.
Hm Hmmmmmmmmm.
Hmmmm Hmmmm.
Hm HMMMMMMM!

This would go on for two minutes every time Mandi brushed. After brushing, Mandi always made sure to go into every nook and cranny between her teeth with floss to make sure her smile was always dazzling.

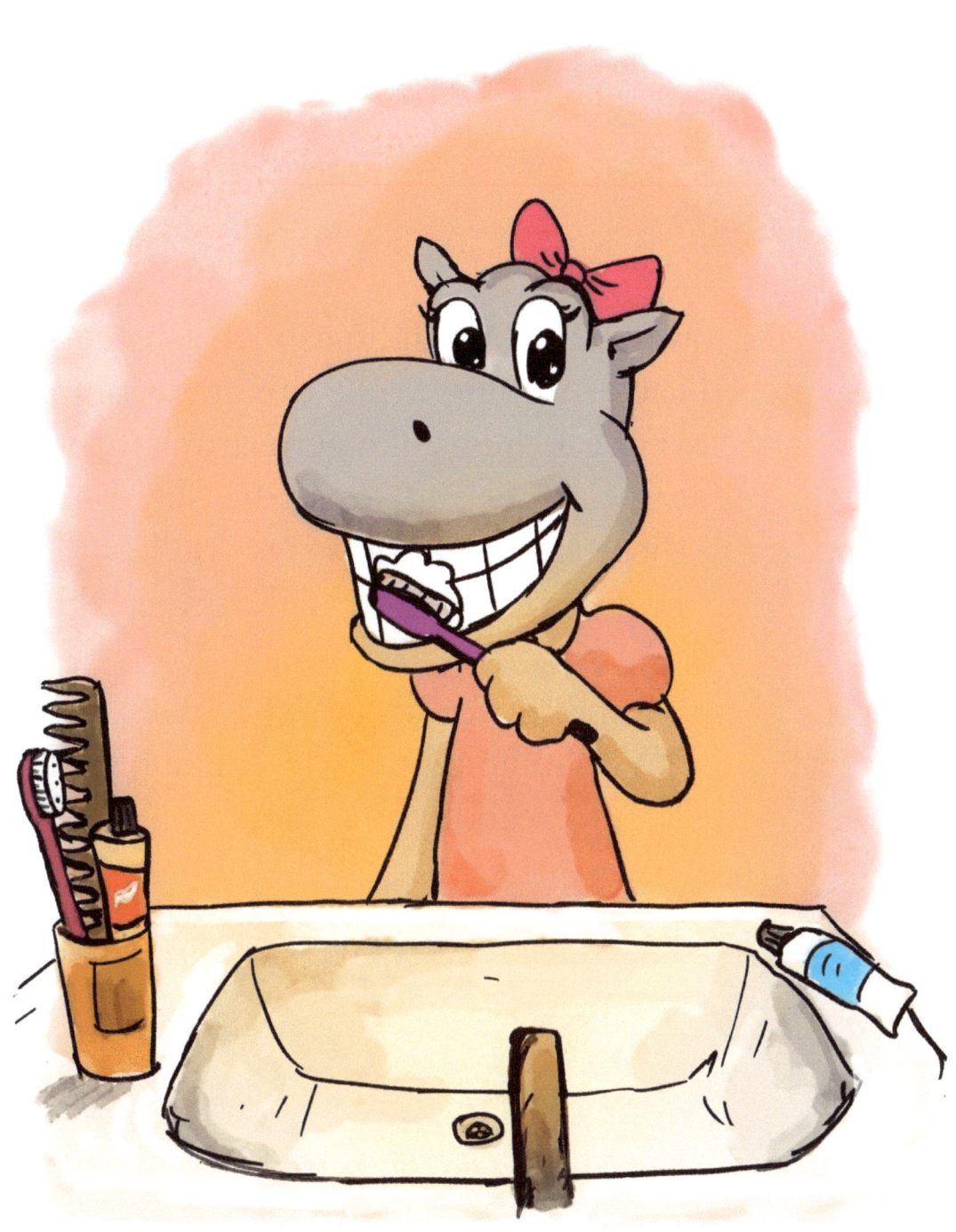

Mandi would always eat fresh grain as well as vegetables that she picked each morning, while the other hippos at school would always eat things like gum drops, Fru-Frus, and cakes of many shapes and sizes. She didn't mind missing out on these sweets, because, as you know, she wanted to make sure her smile was always dazzling.

"If you all keep eating those sweets," she would tell the other hippos, "You're going to end up like old Mr. Peabody!"

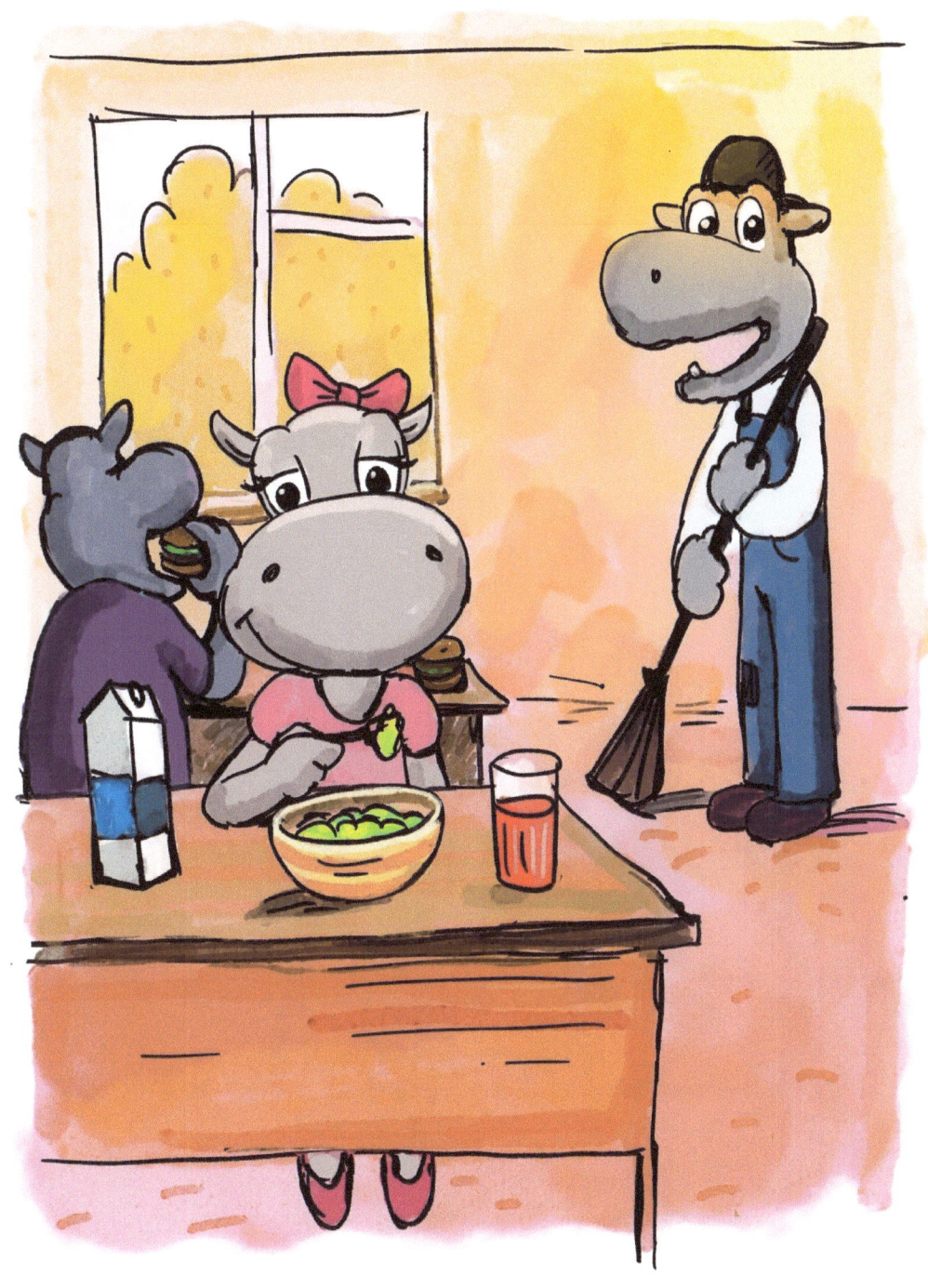

Max, on the other hand, was similar to the other hippos. Every night and every morning while Mandi "Hm Hmm Hmmmmmm'd" with her tooth brush, Max would take a can of the sourest, fizziest soda-pop a hippo can buy and gargle and swish it for two minutes.

Grrgle grrgle gaaaaaaar
Swish swish swish
Gaaaaarrrgle grrgle gurgle.
Swish swish swish

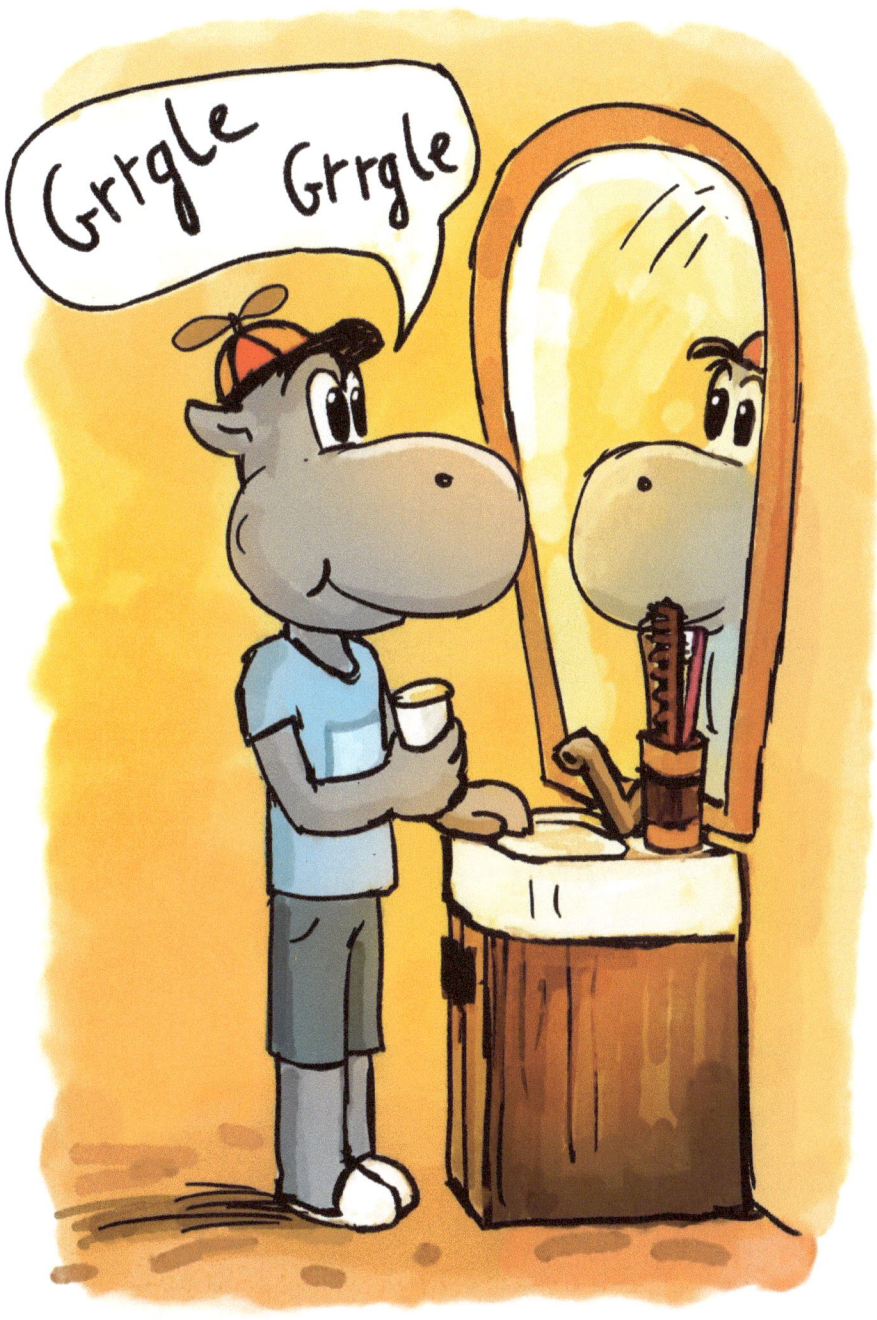

"Mandi, you and I are very alike," Max would say after gargling his soda-pop, "We both take care of our teeth! Only, you put too much effort into it; you should take my advice: all you need to do is swish and gargle soda-pop. The fizz burns those nasty bugs off your teeth with ease!"

"It might take the bugs off your teeth, but don't you see that it also takes your teeth away as well?! If you keep this up, your smile is going to end up like Mr. Peabody's!" Mandi exclaimed.

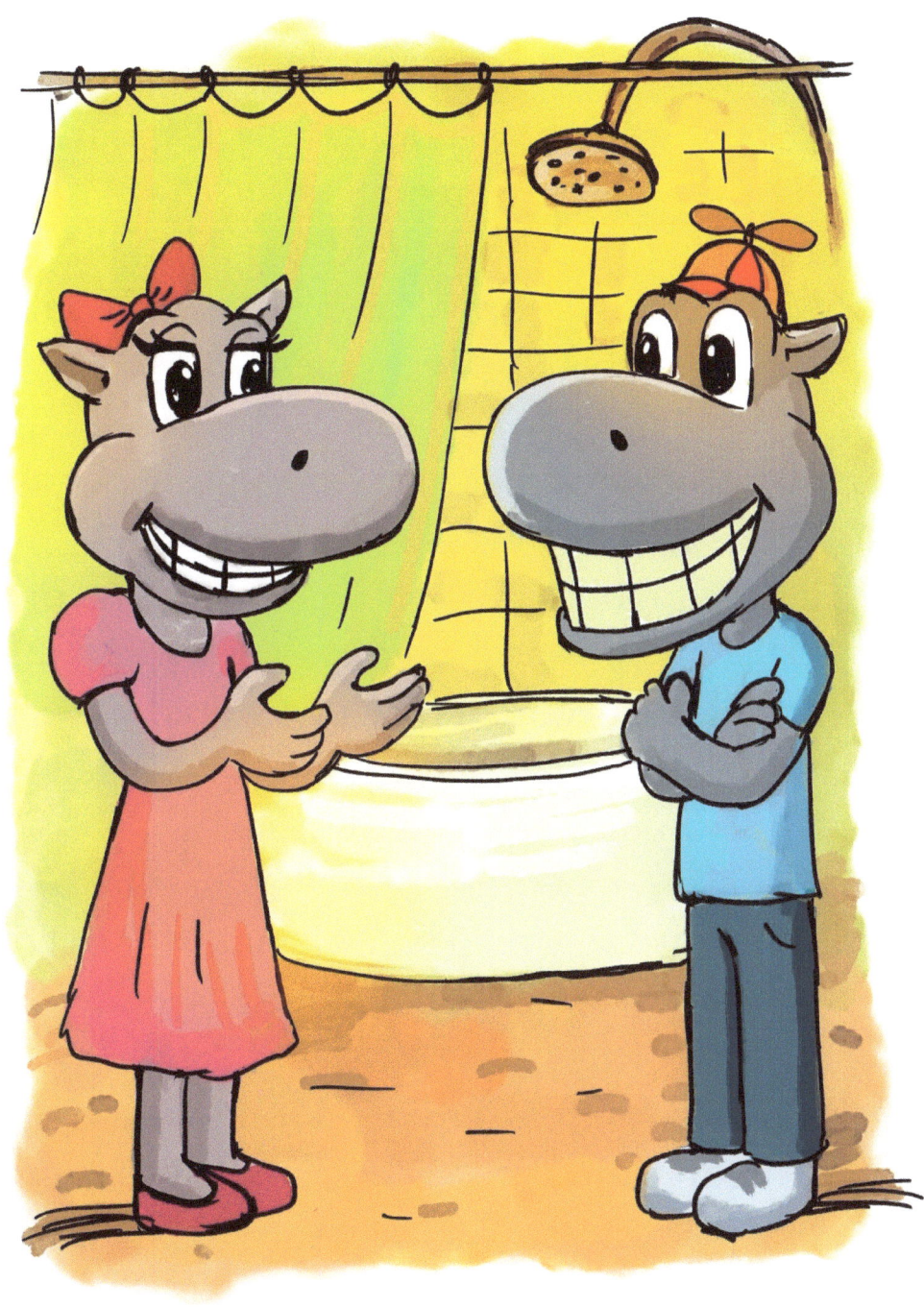

A few short weeks – and a few hundred gum drops, Fru-Frus, and cakes – later, Max began to make a fuss about his mouth hurting.
He looked into the mirror and saw a dark spot on one of his teeth.
"Aiiiieeeeee! This must be the end! To think that I am so young! Mandi, tell all of my loved ones that I will miss them!" Max wailed.

"Don't be ridiculous! Let me see." Mandi said as she looked into Max's mouth.
Mandi saw what looked like a little hole on one of Max's back teeth.
"Ha! What did I tell you? I knew this would happen from you eating all those gum drops, Fru-Frus, cakes, and soda-pop!" Mandi yelled.

"What? That my life would end? Thanks for telling me sooner." Max moaned.

"No, silly! Your tooth has a cavity. Don't worry, though, I read that the traveling dentist Dr. Flo Rhyde is in town today. She's an expert on teeth like ours! Let's go see her!" Mandi said as she dragged Max out of the bathroom.

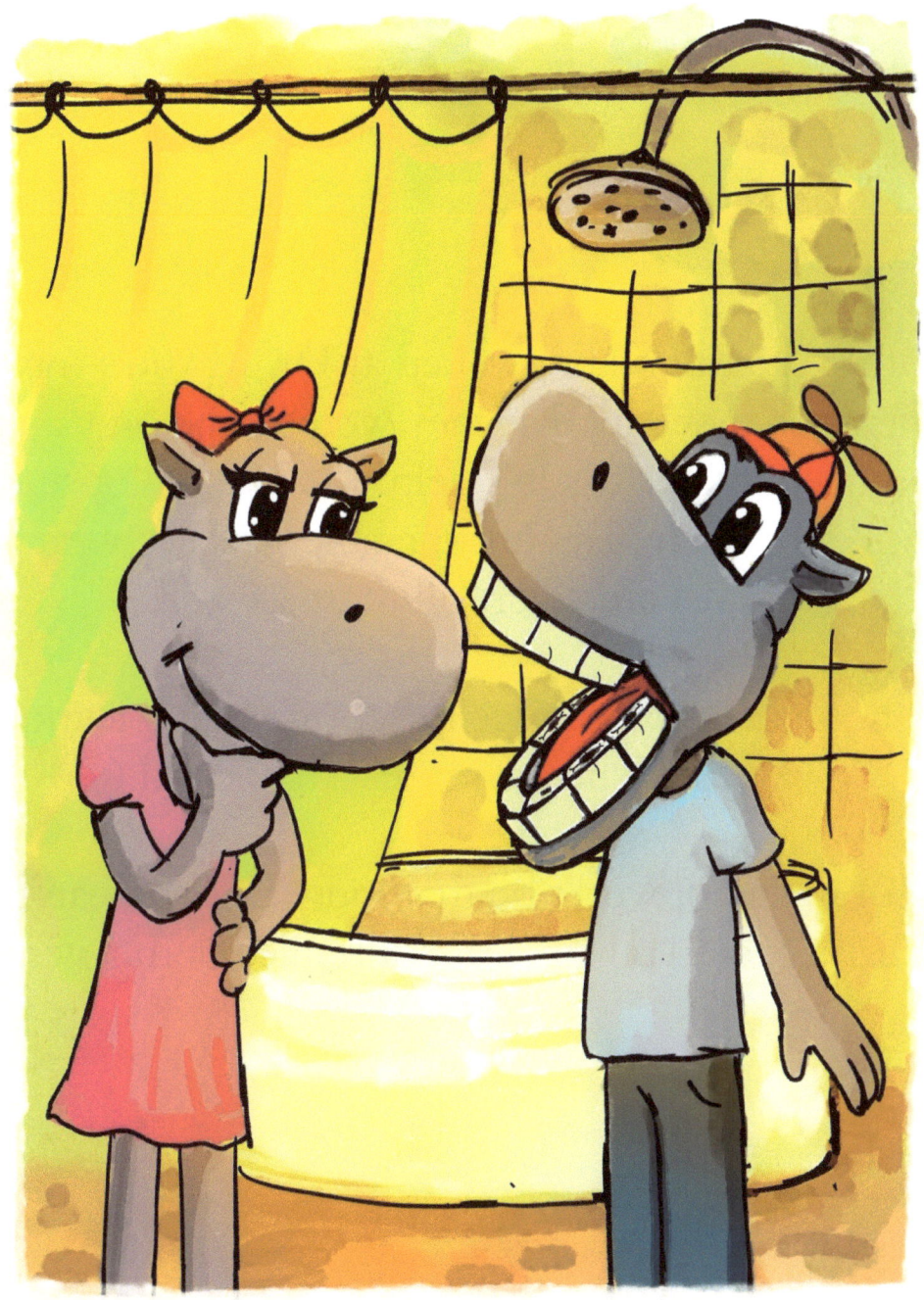

While Max and Mandi waited at Dr. Rhyde's traveling dental bus they saw that they weren't the only animals who needed Dr. Rhyde's help. Lions with loose teeth, monkeys with molars hurting, and gazelles with gums bleeding were all there as well.

"I hope this lady can see me soon! I can't stand this toothache anymore!" Max cried.

"Oh I'm sure it won't be that long! But you can't say I hadn't told you so." Mandi replied with a wink.

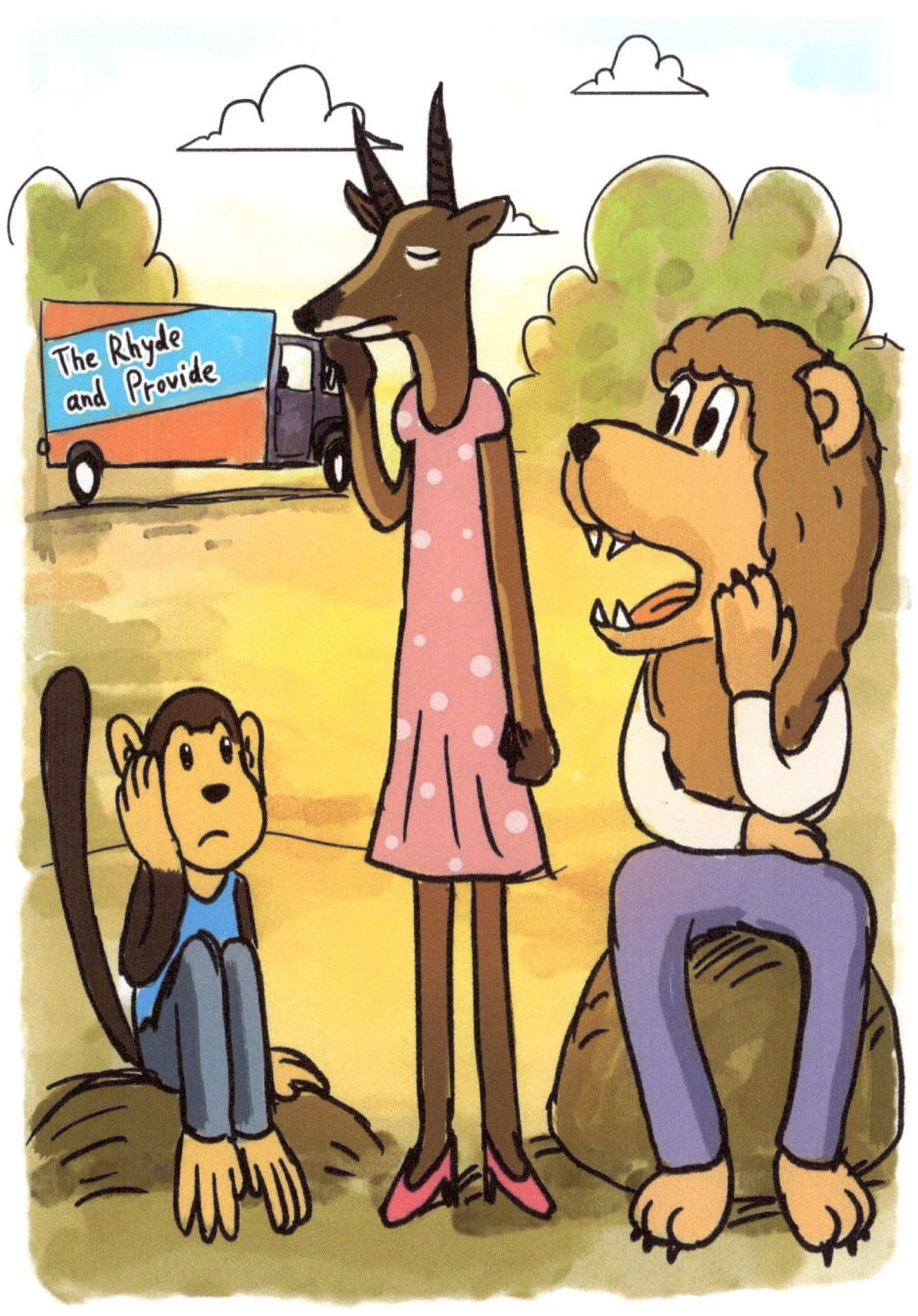

When it was finally Max's turn, Max and Mandi walked onto the bus together.

A voice said "Hello, and welcome to The Rhyde and Provide dental clinic! I'm Dr. Rhyde. What can I do for you two today?"

Max and Mandi first looked left, then they looked right, then they looked in front, then behind, but they could not find out where the voice was coming from. "Down here, you two," said the voice again.

The two hippos looked down and saw two great big yellow eyes staring at them. The lemur smiled as she gave a little wave. "Hello! I'm Dr. Flo Rhyde! What can I do for you two today?"

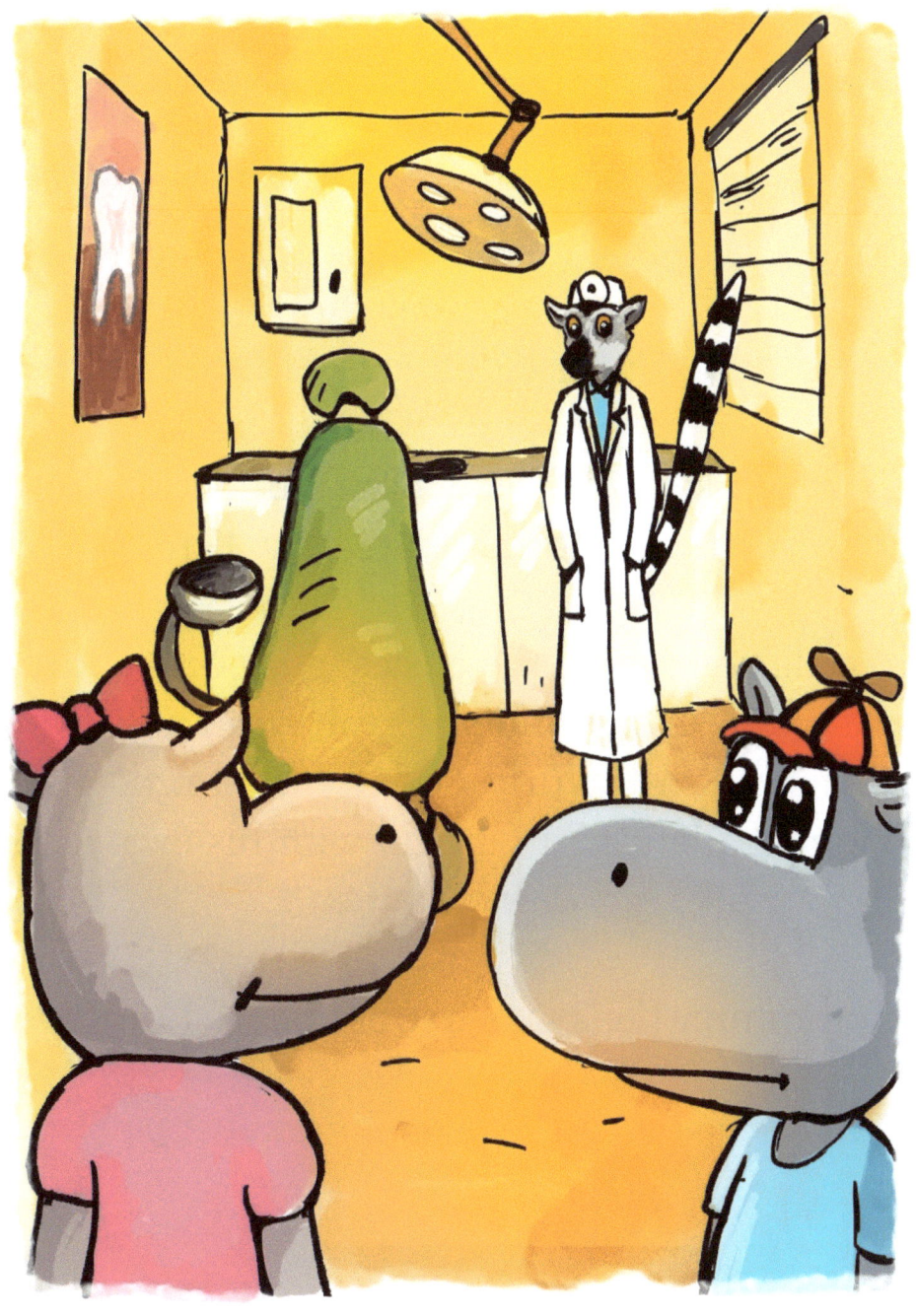

"It's my tooth! It really, terribly, horribly hurts!" Wailed Max. "Please please pleeeeeeeeease help me!"

"Okay, okay, okay – I'll see what I can do. But first, what do you eat on a normal day?" Dr. Rhyde asked.

"Oh, well, you know, the basics: gum drops, Fru-Frus, cakes of many shapes and sizes, oh and I always wash all that down with my favorite soda-pop. MmmMmm how I do so love that stuff." Max said with his eyes the size of dinner plates.

"Hmmmmmm. Let's take a look then." Dr. Rhyde said.

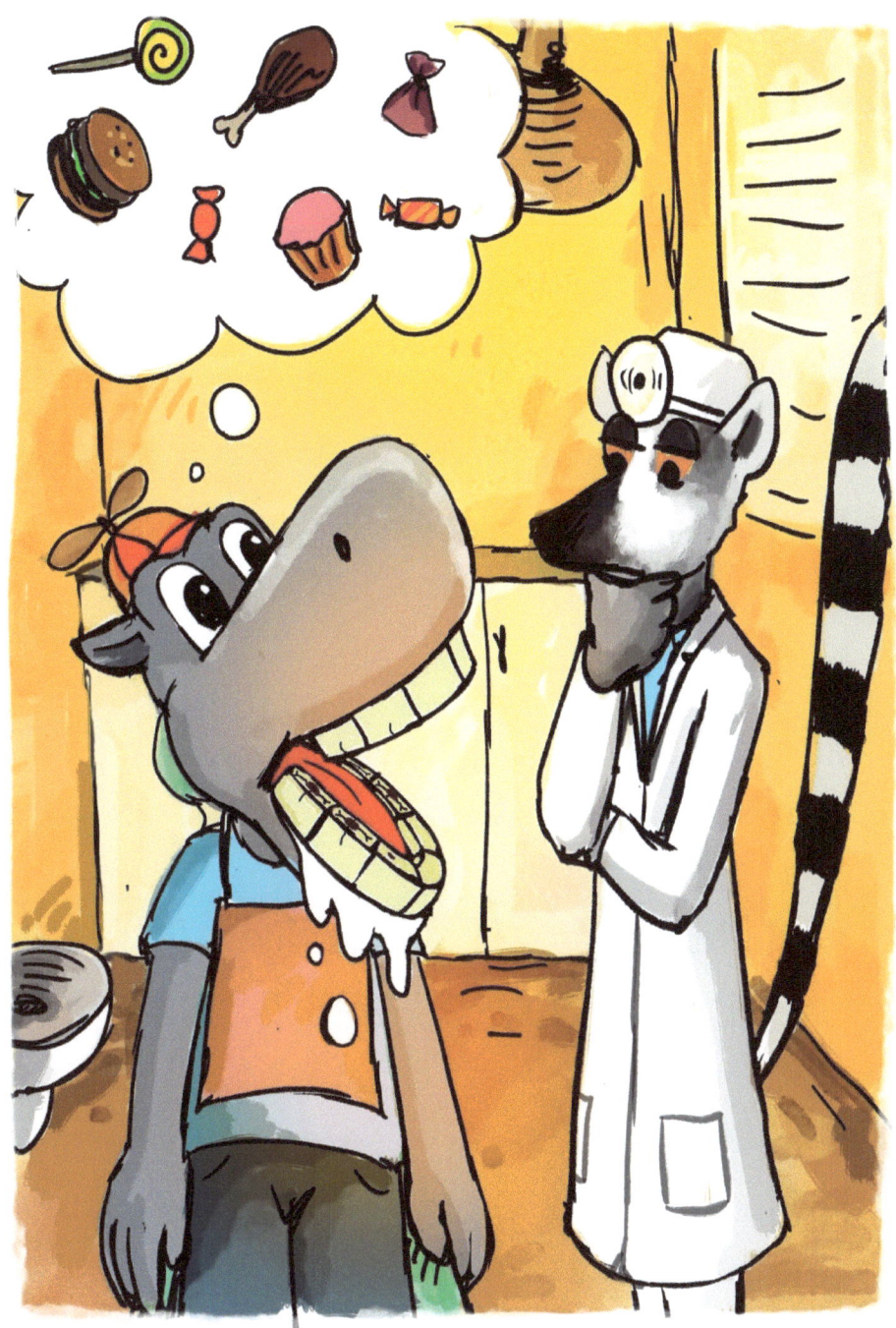

Dr. Rhyde led Max over to her dental chair where she looked into his mouth.

"Well, you do have a cavity, Max, and I can fix that, but I need to tell you something." Dr. Rhyde said as she brought Max up in the chair.

"Eating all the food that you are eating now will cause you to lose those beautiful teeth of yours." Dr. Rhyde said.

"Yeah! I told him he would end up like Mr. Peabody! Mr. Peabody is an old, toothless hippo in this town." Mandi said.

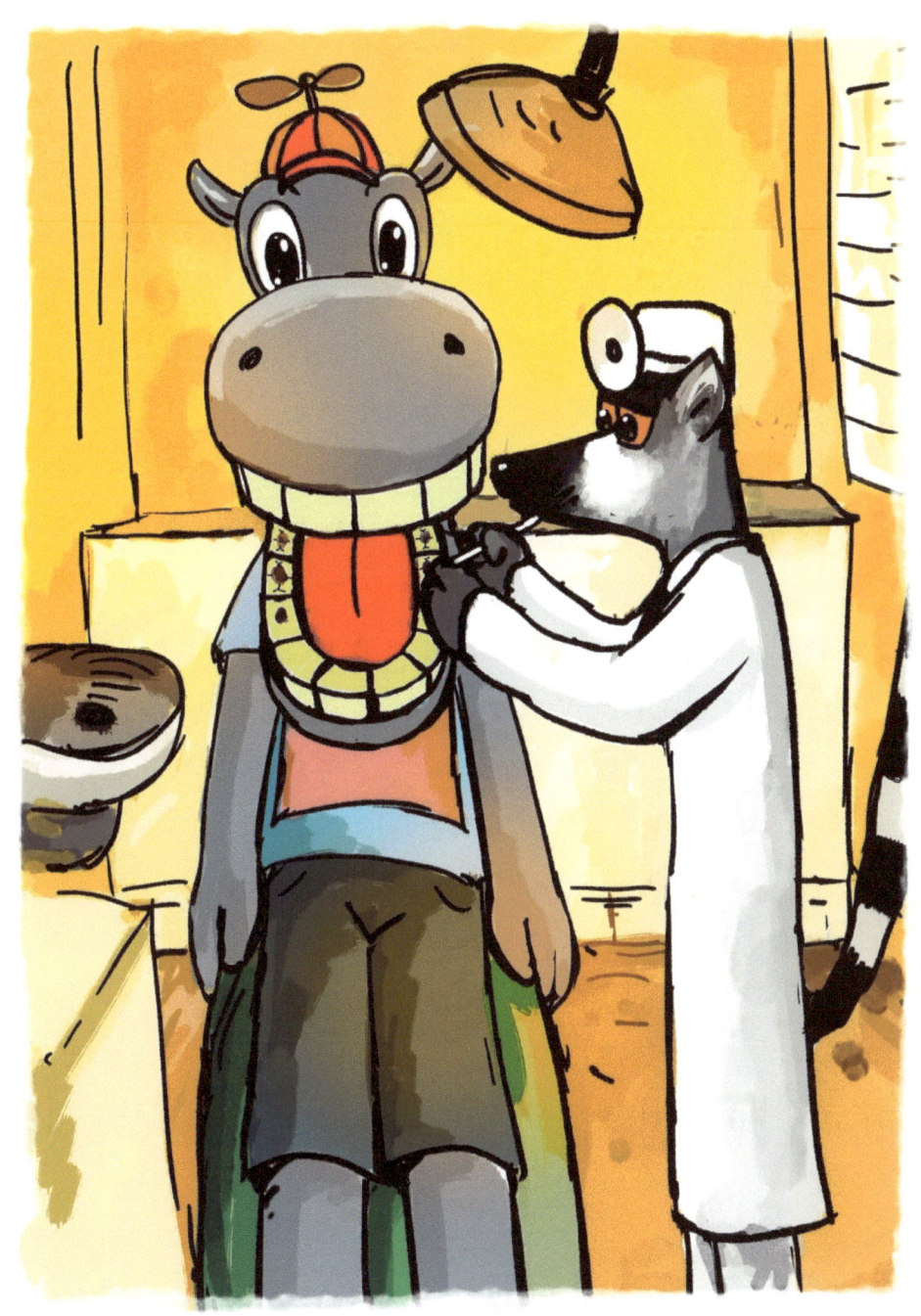

"I don't know about that, but you could lose a lot of them. You need to eat healthy foods, Max, like veggies. What do you do to clean your teeth?" Dr. Rhyde asked Max.

"I gargle some soda-pop. It burns all those nasty bugs off of my teeth!" Max said with pride.

"That's almost true, but did you know that there are bugs that love how sour your soda-pop is?" Dr. Rhyde asked

"No…" Max said as he scratched his head.

"There are! And you're making a home for these bugs to live and hurt your teeth." Dr. Rhyde said

"I had no idea." Max said sadly.

"That's alright! That's why I'm here to help." Dr. Rhyde said. "Let's fix that tooth!"

So after a little this-and-that, Max's tooth was looking good as new.

"Wow, thanks, Dr. Rhyde!" he rejoiced.

"Of course, Max. Just remember what I taught you!" Dr. Rhyde smiled.

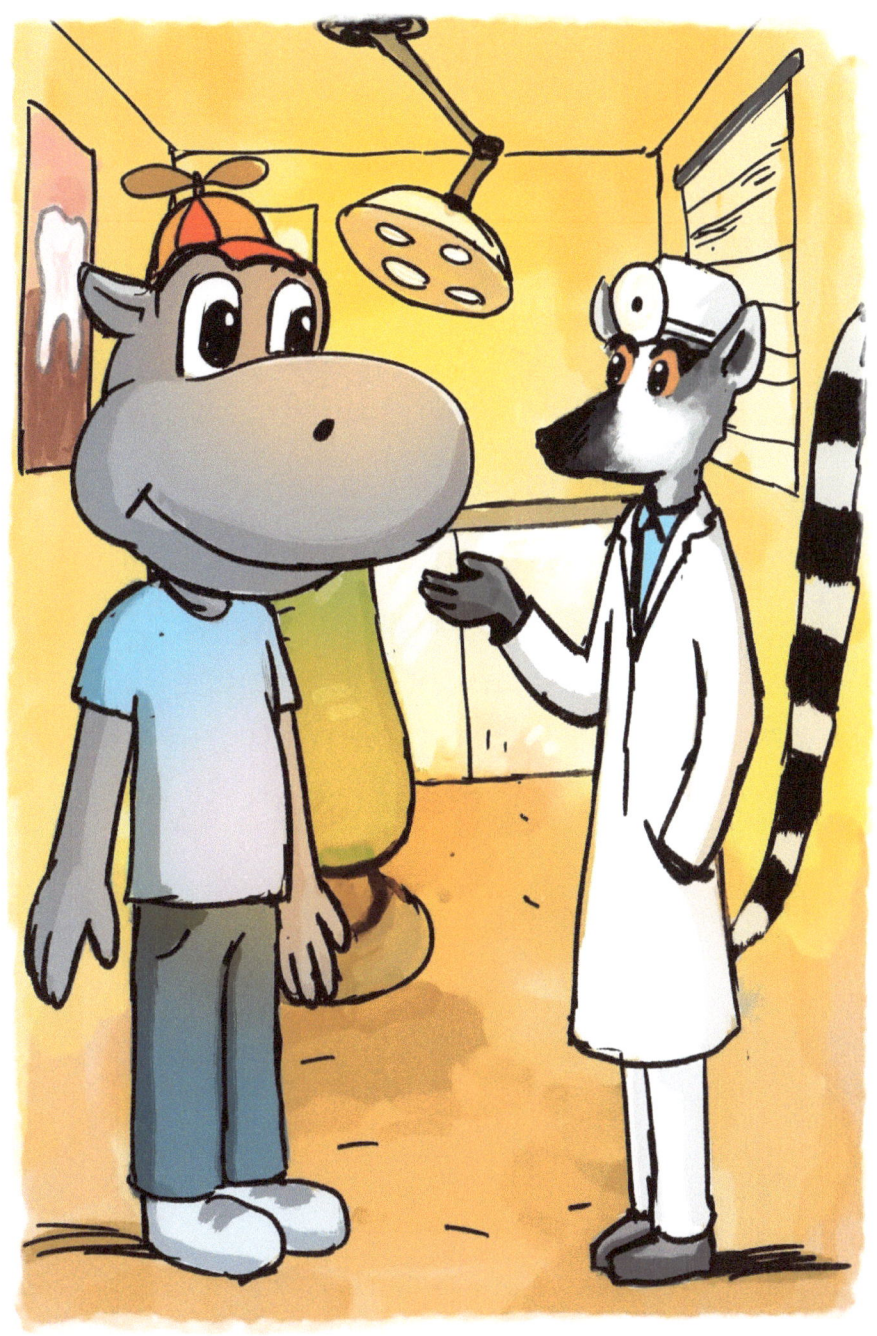

And so, even a year later when Mandi ate her veggies that she picked each morning, and the fresh grain, Max was there doing the same.
And whenever Mandi "Hm Hmm Hmmmmmm'd," Max "Hm Hmm Hmmmmmm'd" back.

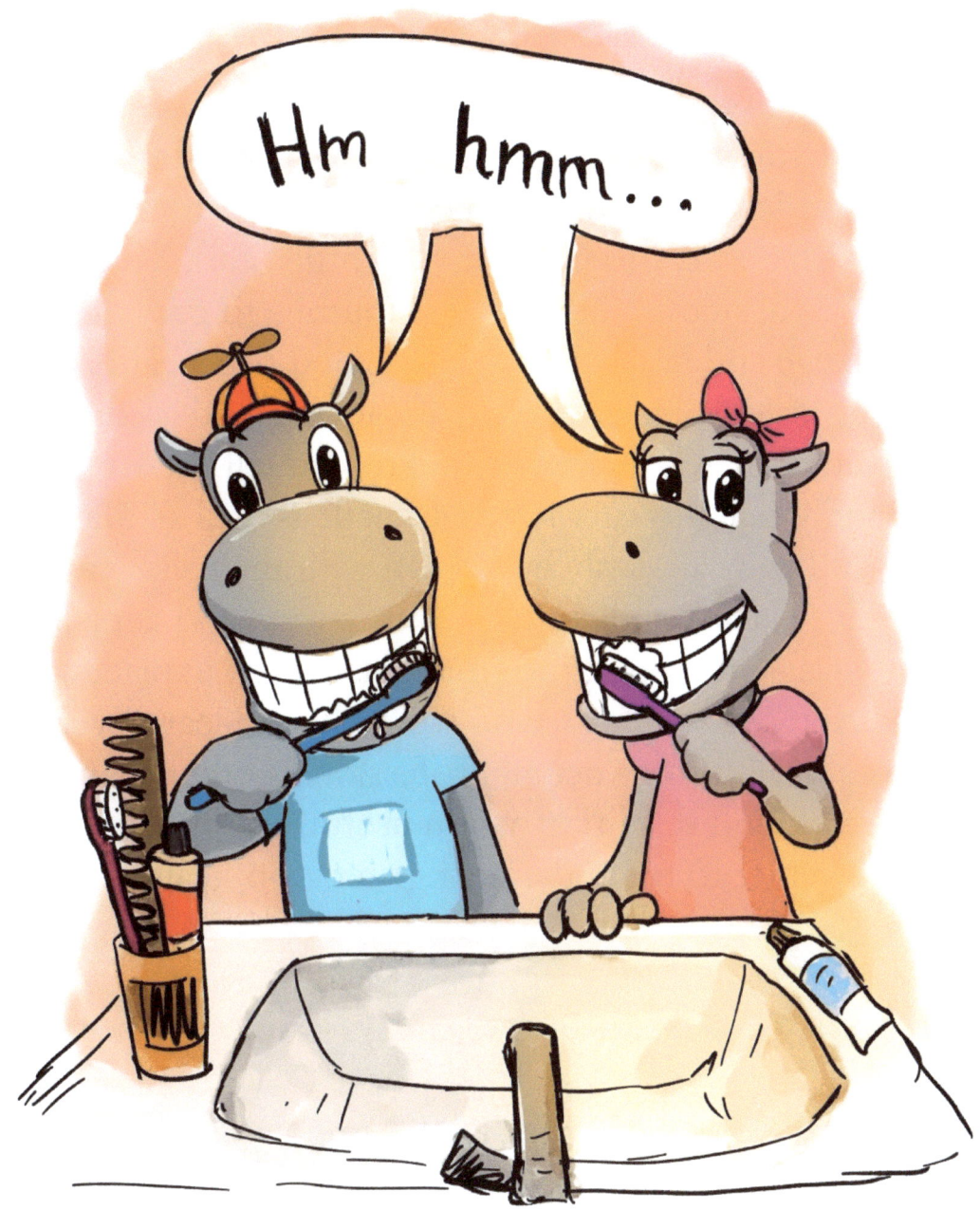

Dear parents and teachers,

First, I want to thank you for picking up this book! Doing so, you have shown that you want to take ownership for your child's/students' oral health. You don't want to just rely on dental professionals to care for your little ones. You want to walk alongside of them on this journey to pass on the knowledge and habits that lead to good oral health. Even though my little story is done, this is not the end of the journey! The children who have listened to you tell the story are hopefully eager to care for their teeth as well as Max and Mandi, and you can easily help them with the following index. Each point corresponds to part of the story, and explains why that part was included in the story. Also, each explanation will include citations for those who would like to learn even more about oral health from dental professionals other than myself. I hope you find this information useful, and that we can all work together to teach the next generation healthy lifelong habits.

Best regards,

Michael T. Nykamp

1. Regarding Mandi's brushing habits:

Many people are unaware of the benefits of brushing one's teeth for two minutes as opposed to the common thirty seconds or less. Brushing one's teeth for two minutes, especially with fluoride toothpaste significantly reduces the risk of tooth decay. Also, brushing one's teeth for two minutes allows for adequate removal of plaque throughout the mouth, reducing the likelihood of gum disease such as gingivitis that could progress to periodontitis.

A. Dijkman, et al. Remineralization of human enamel in situ after 3 months: The effect of not brushing versus the effect of an F dentifrice and an F-free dentifrice. Caries Research: 24(4), 1990.

2. Regarding Mandi's flossing habits:

Quite recently there has been a lot of backlash towards flossing. Regardless of what people may say, flossing by guiding the floss onto each side of the gum tissue between one's teeth – the "C-shaped" technique – is an effective way of removing plaque that a toothbrush's bristles cannot reach. This can help reduce gum disease.

P.P. Hujoel, et al. Dental flossing and interproximal caries: A systematic review. Journal of Dental Research: 85(4), 2006.

3. Regarding the eating habits of the other hippos, and Max's soda-pop swishing:

While these are extreme examples, consuming food and drinks that are high in simple sugars gives the bacteria in one's mouth a lot of nutrients. Although it is true that not all of these bacteria are bad, there are some that take these nutrients, use them, and produce acid as a result. This acid is what leads to tooth decay and cavities. In addition, highly acidic food and drink (i.e. Max's "sourest, fizziest soda-pop") can erode the protective enamel off of one's teeth.

R. Harris, The biology of the children of Hopewood House, Bowral, N.S.W. VI. The pattern of dental caries experience.. Australian Dental Journal: 12(3), 1967

ABOUT THE AUTHOR

Michael Nykamp is a dental student at the University of Michigan School of Dentistry. He lives in Ann Arbor, Michigan with his wife, Alicia. In his spare time, Michael enjoys playing both board and video games, enjoying the outdoors by hiking through forests or walking around Ann Arbor, and occasionally rock climbing as well as other activities. One of Michael's passions is teaching the general public about how they can take care of their health, especially their oral health better.